BEST NUTRITION FOR KIDS

IMPORTANT NUTRITION PARENTS SHOULD GIVE TO THEIR CHILDREN

JOYCE LIFTED

COPYRIGHT

All rights reserved. No part of this publication may be republished in any form or by any means, including translation, scanning, photocopying, etc., without the prior written permission of the copyright owner.

Copyright ©2022 by Joyce Lifted

Table of Contents

INTRODUCTION

Children today tend to eat delicious food,

Most of the foods fall under the category of delicious food rather than high nutritional value.

The category is usually either very sweet or salty.

Tasty selection here is not good for kids at all. However, these foods can be unhealthy. Your child's health may be adversely affected. Some of the problems caused by unhealthy diets can persist into adulthood, even developing into lifelong illnesses.

A healthy diet has many benefits for children which can:

- Stabilize the energy
- Improve their minds
- Balance the mood
- Help them maintain a healthy weight
- Helps prevent mental illnesses such as depression, anxiety and ADHD.

Get all the relevant information here for your child nutrition plan.

CHAPTER ONE

Benefits of Child Nutrition

It is the responsibility of adults to make sure that the meals our children eat for us are like this

As balanced as possible. Children can do this with a balanced diet

Have all the nutrients necessary for an optimal and normal life

Patterns of growth, both mentally and physically. In addition to various

Food groups and supplements that should be included

Food preparation methods should also be part of your child's daily nutrition plan that should be considered to ensure nutritional integrity.

Foundation

Below are some recommendations to consider.

Maintaining a child's nutritional balance, especially in everyday life

Intake: Always provide nutritious snacks such as fresh fruits, vegetables, and yogurt. If your child habitually chooses such nutritious snacks, the potential for unhealthy food choices and intake can have an effect. Will decrease dramatically.

Another good habit to teach your child the importance of reaching for a glass of water rather than sugary drinks.

Water is not only a cheap alternative, but it's also the only completely healthy liquid to consume. .

By sharing nutritious meals with your child as often as possible, simply observing the positive eating habits of adults will encourage your child to make healthy choices. In principle, a child can do this with proper nutrition

Develops mentally and physically without unusual problems.

In both cases, the child's health is also better

As a good foundation for growth and subsequent adulthood

In life.

CHAPTER TWO

Common Nutrient Deficiency

Infant-to-toddler age groups are usually quite limited in the amount of food they can consume. Ensuring that these foods are highly nutritious can be very difficult for adults responsible for a complete and healthy eating plan.

Breastfed infants are said to receive the best, most complete nutrition they need, but most mothers today are unaware of their eating habits and are not sure they are getting the full nutrition they need. They do not ensure adequate nutritional levels.

When this happens, all milk produced is not ideal

Nutritional content. The same is true for childhood age.

The group only provided convenience snacks and groceries.

What is readily available is often not nutritious research.

Nutrients

Below are a unit a number of the defects that area unit seemingly to manifest during a child's health;

- **Calciferol** – common in infants born to vitamin-deficient mothers.

Vitamin D levels in your body system. This is often sometimes

It ends up in the event of hypovitaminosis that could be a weakening of the bones

Sick.

• **Naphthoquinone** - changing into very fashionable

Giving this nutrition to newborns is helpful

It prevents a rare malady that causes neural structure hemorrhage. Iron content – most infants area unit breastfed for her VI months or additional

There is sometimes a risk of developing iron deficiency initial

Year. This will be modified with some extra foods

Diet arrange in addition as relying entirely on breast milk Food. • **Axerophthol** – this is often a fat-soluble nutrient that's hold on in vitamins.

Frequent infections occur once there's Associate in nursing meager quantity of this nutrition within the child's system in step with the requirements of the body and also the body.

CHAPTER THREE

Teach your child to eat healthy

There are many reasons why you should teach your child to eat healthy

From a very early age. By teaching children good eating habits

Daily nutrition program, ensuring all nutrients are taken

The body's needs are well controlled. It also guarantees:

Your child's weight and health will be optimally maintained.

Important Information

Here are some recommendations on how to approach healthy eating for children.

Guidance, not dictation, is how we help children through adoption

Make healthy lifestyle and informed food choices. Provide health

A set of stacks within reach of a child can help in this process

Moreover. Teaching your child to eat more slowly is another way to teach your child good healthy eating habits. By eating slowly, you learn to appreciate and enjoy the food you actually eat.

Involving children in food and shopping is another great way to educate them about the types of healthy foods available and recognize them for their bodily benefits.

Making this exercise as fun and informative as possible will help your child eat healthier in the future. Another good habit to get them involved. This is also another fun way to introduce your child to healthy foods and encourage them to make eating such foods a habit.

Encouraging water consumption over other beverages is another healthy choice to follow. Water not only keeps you hydrated, but is less likely to cause unwanted negative build-up in your body's systems. It is therefore a much better choice.

CHAPTER FOUR

Fighting Childhood Obesity

Most families today have fairly high obesity rates on a family basis. There are many reasons for this, but the most common are lack of exercise and eating very unhealthy foods.

Change food

Below are some recommendations on how to help individuals regain some control and fight obesity;

Maintaining a consistent diet is one way to begin the journey of correcting the negatives of obesity. If a child is accustomed to sticking to specific meal times and strongly discourages eating outside of those times, the child is less likely to seek food outside of the set times. .

This eliminates the need to constantly eat.

Mostly out of habit rather than actually satisfying hunger. Making meals fun and simple is another way to encourage children.

Children enjoy eating. This food party

Fun should also be a child's learning curve.

This does only expands the child's knowledge, but also encourages it a little

A fun way to learn things. They are especially happy that they can show your knowledge to others. This must be upper case upon.

It's also a good idea to lead your child by example, as most children are much attuned to their surroundings and automatically follow what they observe.

By setting a good example while staying healthy, Parenting should do the following;

Parents should be a good model to their children; Youngsters eat the method you eat. Follow the following pointers yourself, and your kids are going to be additional in eating same method too.

Start teaching them young; Food preferences develop early in life.

Expose your kid to different foods early and continue as they grow.

Focus on general nutrition; rather than specializing in specific foods, specialize in your diet. We provide the maximum amount natural food as potential with least process. Avoid prepackaged and processed foods if potential.

Understand what to eat; Abundant of the main target is on what to avoid. This may place you at a drawback. Instead, specialize in what you and your kid ought to eat. This keeps feeding as a positive action.

Don't force them to eat; do not force your kid to "clean the dishes." you have got to be told to pay attention to your body. After you feel full and might stop feeding, you're less possible to overindulge.

Skip meal rewards; after you use food as a gift or to point out heart, your kid could begin mistreatment food to regulate his emotions. Instead, offer hugs, praise, attention, or time spent along.

Limit your screen time; Limiting the number of your time they pay observation TV, computers, or video games will build kids additional possible to seek out one thing additional active. Also, snacking whereas observation TV will cause unconscious feeding, inflicting kids to consume additional calories than they have. I'll have it off.

Set your snack limit; Teach your kid to rise before feeding. Allow them to eat their snacks sitting at the table rather than ahead of the TV. Place snacks like pretzels and popcorn in an exceedingly plate or bowl. Don't enable kids to eat directly from the bag.

Children will come to understand the benefits of fighting obesity and making healthy food choices.

By getting only healthy foods and snacks, your child will become accustomed to these things and will naturally seek them out when needed.

CHAPTER FIVE

Ideal Nutrients for Your Kids

The lifestyle most people adopt today leaves little room for

Make sure a proper diet is followed. This too

Children's nutritionally balanced diet scenario.

Balance

Most people eat on the go or while doing something like mulch

Tasking and kids have learned to break this bad habit.

When this happens, little attention is paid to what is happening

Consumed because the main purpose here is to satisfy hunger.

So when searching, focus first on a more nutritious diet.

The problem is setting many specific times to actually eat.

The entire practice is designed to focus on eating and eating

Process. The next step is to plan your child's nutritional needs according to the highest nutritional value of the foods you choose. Incorporating plenty of fresh fruits and vegetables, especially leafy green varieties, should be emphasized in the diet. .

Eating a Variety of Fruits and Vegetables Keeps You Healthy

Children look forward to cooking. Most of the body

Get Nutrients from a Healthy Supply of Fresh Fruit

And vegetables.

Optimal growth patterns also require protein and carbohydrate consumption, but it should be done in a controlled manner so that a comfortable and healthy balance is achieved. Phytonutrients from these sources produce the required amounts of vitamins C, E, and beta-carotene.

Another important nutrient for optimal child development is

Contains carotenoids including α-carotene, β-carotene,

Lycopene, Lutein, Zeaxanthin, all converted to Vitamin A

Bodily functions. Moderate amount of fluflavonoids

Antioxidants also help maintain arterial and cholesterol levels in children

Visible level.

CHAPTER SIX

Meal Menu for Children

Planning a children's menu can be the most difficult, as children are very picky eaters and seem to prefer meals with little nutritional value. Requires a lot of thought and effort.

Planned

The presence of unhealthiness in the diet is especially true with regard to fried foods where the main unhealthy ingredient in cooking methods is oil.

This type of preparation should be reconsidered whenever possible and alternatives such as broiled, grilled, grilled or served fresh should be chosen.

Colorful foods often resonate with children because children are naturally attracted to foods of different colors. Therefore, the decision to prepare salads as a fast food option is encouraged.

Using plenty of colorful vegetables and fruits,

It is easy on the eyes and has a high nutritional value. Providing light meals

Diet-based is another style to include in your children meal plan.

By having only nutritious snacks available to children, you can minimize the need and sources of unhealthy snacks.

The meal plan also includes a variety of sandwiches, but again color and variety are key. Making sandwiches with low-fat flour and using fillings made from grilled or baked ingredients are better than fried fillings.

Most kids enjoy eating different fillings and substituting one

A traditional tortilla wrap sandwich would be interesting

An innovative way to add items to your menu. Using other healthy wraps should also be part of your meal plan, and these may include simple ingredients such as cabbage leaves and different types of flatbreads.

CHAPTER SEVEN

Fundamental Nutrients and Minerals for Youngsters

Below are some recommendations for essential vitamins and minerals that should ideally be part of your child's nutrition plan.

Vitamin

Calcium - Necessary for healthy bones and teeth

Sufficient levels of calcium in the body at all times. Growing

Children need this element to ensure optimal growth.

Calcium can be also being gotten from consumption of milk, dairy products, spinach, kale, etc.

Almond

Iron - Iron keeps your blood healthy and improves the flow of oxygen to your tissues. A lack of iron in the body can lead to anemia, which can have many negative effects on children. Iron can be obtained from red meat, beans, and iron fortifying foods such as: B. Found in certain grains.

Magnesium - This mineral is used to keep your heart beating healthy

It also builds a strong immune system and strong bones. For

Growing children, this is an important factor to ensure that

Since these age groups tend to have large bellies,

Falls and minor accidents are more common than other age groups. Good source

Magnesium is found in whole grains, fish, nuts, potatoes, and dairy products.

Product.

Potassium - This is another important factor required for proper development of optimal bodily functions. These include renal development and blood pressure status. Potatoes, bananas, avocados, and fish are good sources of potassium.

Then there is a list of vitamins that are also useful for various other vitamins

Not only does the child's body cope well with defenses, but it's potential

Achieve optimal mental and spiritual growth, not just illness

Physically.

CHAPTER EIGHT

Instructions to Defeat Dietary problem

Most eating disorders are caused by simple negligence or negligence.

Uninformed upbringing or overzealous eating habits. Everyone

Or a combination of these can seriously affect the big picture

Healthy growth of children. Ideally there should be some guidelines on how to do this

Helping Young and Inexperienced Parents Recognize and Cope this responsibility.

Things necessary

There are three main types of eating disorders: pica, rumination disorder, and childhood or early childhood eating disorders. Pica focuses on the consumption of non-food items such as hazardous materials and toys. Rumination disorder is a chronic eating disorder.

Regurgitation of ingested food but not severe enough to be classified

As vomiting. Finally, there are eating disorders in infancy.

Malnutrition in childhood and here

Medical problem.

There are some recommendations that can and should be followed in order to properly deal with this issue.

If you follow these recommendations carefully, you can even reverse your eating disorder and help your child adjust to normal eating habits. More socially acceptable.

Increased Calories, Minerals, Vitamins, Quantity

The water your child consumes is one way to keep them more engaged.

A balanced and acceptable meal plan. Make sure your food is presented

With attractive designs and versatility, it also encourages the child's cooperation to participate in the meals provided. Trying to identify the presence of a medical condition that may contribute to the eating disorder is another method that can be taken to solve the problem of eating disorders.

CHAPTER NINE

THE RIGHT NUTRIENTS FOR THE KIDS

A simple technique for guaranteeing that children get the nutrients they have is by choosing quality food sources for them to eat.

Pick lean macromolecule from sources like poultry, beans, fish, nuts, and seeds.

Eat new, canned, or frozen veggies foods systematically. search around for canned and frozen selections while not other fats or sugars. Natural merchandise have to be compelled to be in 100% or water.

Pick entire grain food varieties like bread, cereals, and food that are high in fiber.

Search for low-fat dairies like milk, cheddar, and dairy product for grown-ups and children in your loved ones. Youngsters should not have farm things until they are one year recent. The Yankee Institute of medicine prescribes entire milk for youngsters twelve to 2 years, except if your baby is deed excess weight. Inquire on whether or not you do not grasp.

It's likewise important to limit other and refined sugars, refined grains, sodium, trans, fats, immersed fats, and food sources that are low in supplements.

Nutrition are significant, however, segment size matters as well.

A big part of your kid's plate ought to be foods grown from the ground.

Pick new food varieties over profoundly handled food varieties.

What you cook and plan food sources can mean the dietary benefit. For instance, have a go at barbecuing, steaming, baking, or cooking vegetables as opposed to searing or bubbling them.

It's not simply food that is significant. Hydrate or low-fat milk rather than sweet, improved drinks.

Various food varieties give various supplements, so ensure your kid gets a decent assortment of leafy foods.

IN CONCLUSION

Having a healthy child is every parent's desire to be healthy.

Children are happy children and visits to the doctor

Very costly and stressful

Sum of.

www.ingramcontent.com/pod-product-compliance
Lightning Source LLC
LaVergne TN
LVHW020531160826
845677LV00015B/4005

* 9 7 9 8 3 7 0 8 8 0 7 2 8 *